# 50 BUSINESS IDEAS
## FOR HEALTH CARE
### PROFESSIONALS

# 50 BUSINESS IDEAS FOR HEALTH CARE PROFESSIONALS

A GUIDE FOR HEALTH CARE BUSINESS OWNERSHIP

Eva M. Francis, RN, MSN, CCRN

ISBN: 1522862188
ISBN 13: 9781522862185

# INTRODUCTION

This is a book that will change the lives of Health Care professionals—or any other smart, highly motivated individuals—who are passionate about taking their personal and professional lives to the next level of success. If you are a Health Care professional or anyone else who feels ready to make the move by starting your own business, but you are not sure what it is that you are passionate about or how to proceed, this book is definitely a "must-have" for you as you take on this amazing journey of "pursuing your life's purpose". This book is for you if you are seeking to change the lives of those you come in contact with on a regular basis.

This book will give you clarity as you embrace your passion and do what you love to do best. When I wrote this book, I had in mind Health Care professionals who have been at the bedside or in the clinical area and want to make a change or a shift with service as the core. I believe that service is the key to greatness. I also thought about the nurses who have navigated their way from the bedside to the boardroom and now want to go beyond the boardroom—this book is for you and will give you insights into your dreams and aspirations. There are so many alternatives for nurses or for health care professionals to reinvent and re-tool their lives .Being a business owner and an entrepreneur will take you through a journey of self discovery and does not mean that you are not serving others, especially patients. In fact, as a business owner and an entrepreneur, you will have the power, the flexibility  and the opportunity to be more, do more, and serve more. You will have the power to shift the direction of processes and launch new discoveries as you unveil new things every day within yourself as well as in Health care. Whether you touch the lives of people directly or indirectly, you will be changing lives constantly. There is no better way to serve than giving of your time to those who are vulnerable and need your service. So enjoy this book and have fun elevating and upgrading your life, career, and your profession.

# Disclaimer

All the material contained in this book is provided for educational and informational purposes only. No responsibility can be taken for any results or outcomes resulting from the use of this material.

While every attempt has been made to provide information that is both accurate and effective, the author does not assume any responsibility for the accuracy or use/misuse of this information.

# TABLE OF CONTENTS

# CHAPTER 1

## CONTINUING HEALTH CARE INDUSTRY CHANGES: IMPACT ON THE NURSING PROFESSION

The Health Care system is ever changing, especially over the last decade. Many people are becoming increasingly health conscious day by day, but some individuals face life threatening situations in cases of malignant or chronic disease. There have been transitions for those in nursing and other allied professions. The industry has promised to change the practice of Health Care, expand upon current roles, make room for new Health Care practices, and provide increased opportunities for nurses and allied health practitioners to participate in molding the future delivery system for Health Care. In short, the Health Care industry is facing unprecedented challenges, and as Health Care professionals we must brace ourselves to play a major role in meeting these demands. The medical profession is the supreme profession in the history of all professions in this world. No health disorder could be prevented or cured without the knowledge that the health sector provides. Through medical research we now know that numerous diseases are feeding into each other. For example, in some underdeveloped countries, goiter is a common disorder that can happen because of either a genetic problem or a deficiency in dietary iodine. If goiter isn't treated properly, this deficiency may cause serious issues, including diabetes, mental retardation, and growth deficiency.

Since the Affordable Care Act (ACA) was passed in 2010, care delivery and financing systems have been undergoing major changes that are continuing to accelerate. Due to the ACA, millions more Americans have, and are going to continue to gain, health insurance. This shift will require a sizable workforce to meet the increased demand for care. This increased demand for care is in turn, causing the Health Care workforce to face increased stress and instability . This is due to a major shift in the different types of Health Care providers that are needed to accommodate the services needed for millions more Americans. One goal that stems from the ACA is enhanced coverage for preventative-care services, shifting away from the current focus of the delivery system on acute care. There needs to be a greater emphasis on prevention and treatment of chronic conditions using Health Care teams along with information technology. This shift in focus could help disseminate valuable health-related news and information to those who are working with patients. This is major, especially for those of us who are passionate about taking Health Care to another level and launching our own businesses.

With the continuing advancements of technology and the aging human population, the challenges that nurses face are not getting easier, as some may think. The health conditions that individuals are being diagnosed with are more frequently chronic, requiring a longer duration of treatment, and requiring adjustments in treatment according to any unfamiliar route the condition decides to take. As a consequence, nurses need ongoing education to stay abreast of new treatments, as well as new diseases. We frequently hear about new strains of illnesses surfacing or diseases that are becoming resistant to current treatments because of unrestricted antibiotic use—without acknowledgment of the harm of overdoses of vaccines or antibiotics. This requires the nursing profession to break out of its comfort zone and come up with new ways to provide treatment and care. Some nurses may even opt to continue their education so that they may increase their level of practice for certain situations, and many times they become as knowledgeable as general physicians in these areas.

Another impact that the ever-changing Health Care industry may have on the nursing profession is causing shortages of medical professionals, most predominantly in rural areas. Along with an aging population, we also have an aging workforce that is going to cause hundreds of thousands—or even millions—of job openings for nurses and physicians within the next five years. With the numerous new additions to the medical profession, there will be new attitudes toward professional roles and responsibilities that differ from those that the prior generation held. Based on the current situation that is unfolding, it seems likely that there will not be enough licensed nursing professionals in the United States to take care of the number of Americans needing care. This is scary to think about. If there are not enough professionals to handle the aging population and their chronic conditions, there may be an increase in morbidity and mortality, especially for rural elders. They would be more vulnerable to the spread of fatal disease by water, air, and food. In addition, this population tends to have poor medical centers in the surrounding areas, and as a result the risk is growing. A shortage of medical personnel and possible increases in mortality would defeat the goal of increasing the average life span of rural people, who deserve the same services as modern city dwellers.

More and more newly insured patients entering into the Health Care setting means a heavier workload for the professionals who take care of them. In turn, this results in more stress, more paperwork, longer hours, more errors, and higher levels of fatigue. Ultimately, some Health Care providers will become burned out or second-guess their career decisions. I suppose the optimistic person would say that there is only one way to go from the current Health Care industry situation, and that is up! However, to push past the long hours, heavy workloads, prolonged dissatisfaction, and increased stress, one must be stretched to the limit and be 100 percent passionate about this career. It always seems like if you stick with something long enough, the positive aura of it shines through sooner or later.

Year after year, advancement after advancement, we all have to do our very best to accept change in the Health Care industry and hope that the kinks work themselves out. The majority of the changes that we are seeing can ultimately be beneficial if carried out correctly, especially in medicine and nursing. Embrace the changes as best as you possibly can, because they could mean a cure for your disease or a few more years to spend with those you love.

# CHAPTER 2

## WHY HEALTH CARE ENTREPRENEURSHIP?

In today's Health Care industry, there have been some notable changes taking place, and an equal number of entrepreneurial opportunities and activities have arisen as a direct response. Health Care is a trillion-dollar business and governments around the world have increased spending on Health Care. Individuals understand that Health Care is not a luxury but an obligation of the government. But, even so, the authorities won't always be capable of providing sufficient health service to everyone. In 2014 alone, there was a vast increase in the number of start-ups involved in the Health Care industry. For example, Omada Health is a company that connects those at risk for chronic diseases such as type 2 diabetes to a comprehensive lifestyle-change program that includes a personal health coach and a digital support group. There is a wealth of support for entrepreneurs who are developing new solutions to address some of the growing pains in Health Care.

Entrepreneurs involved in the Health Care industry help aid the current providers of Health Care services by introducing innovative technologies that, in many cases, make it easier to do their jobs. This, however, does not mean that becoming an entrepreneur in the Health Care industry is easy. Entrepreneurship in any industry is not easy, and not everyone is suited to becoming an entrepreneur. However, there are many reasons to consider becoming an entrepreneur. Here are some reasons to become an entrepreneur who focuses on the Health Care sector:

- **Increased investment.** One of the main reasons entrepreneurs should consider Health Care entrepreneurship is the amount of funds that venture capitalists are pumping into the sector. As previously stated, there has been a record increase in the amount of money that start-ups are receiving for ideas.
- **Opportunity.** There are plenty of opportunities involved in the Health Care industry, which can help explain why there is so much revenue being pumped into it. Physicians and nurses with practical experience have new avenues for their expertise.
- **Social Responsibility.** Some of the opportunities that are present in the Health Care industry are a result of many medical practitioners' and other entrepreneurs' commitment to help build and improve their society.
- **Create Smiles.** The most successful entrepreneurs are the ones whose first goal is to make a difference and add value to the lives of others, as opposed to making money. The Health Care industry is one of the best places that entrepreneurs can do something to help effect real change in people's lives and create smiles on their faces. In many cases, when the primary objective of an entrepreneurial undertaking is to effect positive change, money and financial freedom follow.

Often in the Health Care industry, doctors and other practitioners are the ones getting involved in entrepreneurship, but savvy entrepreneurs who are not doctors are normally able to identify the opportunities involved and take advantage of them as well. Health Care is becoming and will remain a great opportunity hub for entrepreneurship for a long time. It is estimated that in 2015 more Health Care start-ups will emerge, and more venture capitalists will invest more money in these companies. The time for Health Care entrepreneurship is now, and more smart entrepreneurs will indeed be getting involved in this industry.

Along your journey, keep in mind the **SEVEN TIPS** that follow so that you can aspire to be the best you can be in whichever Health Care entrepreneurial opportunity you jump into headfirst.

- **1. Understand the "WHY" behind your aspiration.** You must always remain confident in your skills and experiences and never falter when asked questions about why you choose such a career path. Individuals like to see that they are being led by a strong-minded person who knows exactly what he or she wants and how to get it. I learned long ago that if your "why" is strong enough, you do not need to worry about the "how." Your why must be in alignment to a greater cause, and actually greater than yourself.

- **2. Be knowledgeable about your business. We all know that knowledge is power.** A business needs to be led by an entrepreneur who is always professional, who knows the business's values by heart, and who does not underestimate how much work is involved in enabling the business to run smoothly and to grow on a daily basis. Being knowledgeable about the organization does not happen overnight; it is a process that comes with consistency and patience. Knowledge comes through involving yourself in the business 24/7 at whatever cost, gaining new experience over time, and always being the go-to person that others can turn to in times of need. Entrepreneurs should believe in themselves, be confident in the journey, and expect to succeed in whatever they are doing. They also must have just as much knowledge about their entrepreneurship workforce and their industry.

- **3. Be knowledgeable about the Health Care industry.** Whenever an entrepreneur is willing to launch a business in the Health Care arena, he or she needs to bear in mind that the primary goal is to serve needy people facing untreated disease. Service is key. Continually building upon your knowledge regarding the Health Care arena is very important because it changes frequently. You must be able to be flexible within the ever-changing medical field and always be open to learning new things. Remember that the Health Care knowledge you gain should also be shared with others within your organization in order to keep business practices up to date and to provide the best services possible.

- **4. Demonstrate success—always.** A successful entrepreneur should always be a role model for others, not only to look up to but also to trust without any doubt. You should demonstrate success while in the workplace at all times, to the best of your ability. Never pass up a chance to help others along the way; you want to avoid burning any bridges.

- **5. Develop leaders.** Professionals in business should always do their best to surround themselves with successful and optimistic people who share the same values and aspirations. In this way, the entire team can serve as professional, successful leaders in their positions.

- **6. Network with influencers.** Professionals should always network, or be a part of groups, in order to stay motivated and determined. Negativity should never be tolerated.

7. **Aspire to perform only at professional standards—nothing less!** Professionalism and ethics are critically important within the Health Care profession. One must be aware of one's own beliefs before being able to handle the problems others may be facing. Successful entrepreneurs should assume professionalism in all aspects of life. They must *never* bring a personal problem to work. Professionalism is essential, and the public expects nothing less. Especially when you are in the medical field, professionalism must be demonstrated to the sick and injured.

# CHAPTER 3

## FIFTY BUSINESS IDEAS FOR HEALTH CARE PROFESSIONALS

- **For Health Care professionals who are interested in being independent—rather than sitting around and waiting for their next paycheck for working in hospitals or various designated organizations—here are fifty ideas on how to be self-employed as a health care entrepreneur.**

1. **Health Care Directorial Consultant**—Those who become health-and-wellness treatment consultants are people who have a passion to aid wellness-treatment companies run successfully, sensibly, and with the foremost objective of guaranteeing people safety and security. In addition to a passion for this area, health-and-wellness treatment experts need an education and experience in company or wellness-treatment management. The educational requirement may differ based on clients and employers; however, a master's degree in a relevant field may be required. Income may vary as well and may depend on factors such as experience and duties. This can be a very fulfilling field for those looking for independence and wanting to build a practice to work for themselves.

2. **Professional Health Care Speaker**—Health Care practitioners with years of experience in Health Care, or with expertise in some aspect that people are willing to learn more about, can set up a speaking practice. When a Health Care practitioner counsels or advises patients, the good counsel may be 50 percent of the cure. Share your expertise and skills with people at conferences and workshops, and get paid for this. You will need to have expertise in an area to be able to speak about it, and the fees will vary depending on the type of speaking engagement. One can increase and sharpen and crystallize their speaking and presentation skills by joining their local toastmasters group which is a very low cost to join.

3. **Health Care Motivational Speaker**—Do you have a passion for interesting people in their health and boosting their morale, or do you have a passion for educating the masses about the Health Care system? If you do, then this may be a career for you. You get paid to motivate people to action by speaking to them at seminars, workshops, and conferences. Nowadays, there are many enthusiastic nurses who have a lot of years of experience. These experts can easily establish themselves as senior motivational speakers in the Health Care arena. Though special qualifications for this job may vary, you will need to have a love for what you do and be able to motivate people You will also need excellent speechwriting and public-speaking skills. I remember when we were planning our first "Nurse Empowerment Summit." We were looking for a motivational speaker who would be able to inspire and motivate the audience. To my surprise, this task was extremely difficult. We could not find Health Care speakers who were also motivating and empowering. I am not

saying that they don't exist, but clearly there is a need for more inspirational and motivational speakers in this area. This is a business venture that would make such a difference. If you like public speaking, this is for you. There are many ways to improve your public speaking skills to get this type of business up and running. My recommendation is to start improving your skills by joining Toastmasters International. There are many local groups around the country and it is extremely inexpensive to join. Not only will participation in Toastmasters increase and improve your speaking skills, but it will definitely also improve your leadership skills. This is vital when you are getting ready to launch a new business.

4.  **Health Care Holistic Coach**—Maybe you have a passion for helping people increase vitality, decrease stress, and sculpt the body of their dreams. If so, you may consider becoming a holistic lifestyle coach. This position would allow you to show people how disease and stress are preventable through healthy eating habits, lifestyle management, and appropriate types of exercise. Many people pay these coaches top dollar since people are more conscious of their health today.

5.  **Health-and-Wellness Coach**—As a health-and-wellness coach, you will help your clients find the motivation and tools to achieve physical and emotional health goals. You will help clients make better choices that fit their lifestyles. Some goals that your clients may have include the following:
    a.  Decrease obesity, especially morbid obesity
    b.  Improve diet
    c.  Quit smoking

    d.   Lower stress, without taking stress-relieving drugs

    e.   Overall lifestyle improvement

    If this sounds like something you're interested in, then this may be a great option for you. Again, your earning potential will depend on your passion, your clients, and your services.

6.  **Integrative Health Coach**—As an integrative health coach, you will coach clients to develop and engage in healthy mind-sets and behaviors. Using evidence-based theories and practices, you will assist clients in improving their health and well-being through personal responsibility and self-motivation. You may need to have some certification—whether it be a certificate as an integrative health coach or in a related field. This is a great option, and again, earning potential depends on your clientele and exactly what you will be doing with those clients.

7.  **Legal Health Care Consultancy Business**—Use your expertise as a medical practitioner and provide expert advice to lawyers and other legal professionals on matters in the Health Care industry. To get involved in this business, you will need to have experience and expertise in a particular field, as well as any required qualifications for that field. If you meet the requirements, then this can be a great option for you, and—like other consulting practices—the earning potential will vary.

8.  **Health-and-Fitness Coach**—This is one of the most popular routes that someone can take to get involved in the Health Care industry. If you have a passion for helping people live a healthy lifestyle, if you want to teach people about the amazing human body and what it is capable

of, and if you would like to guide people to the right exercises to do in order to stay physically fit and enjoy good health, then this is the job for you. Again, you will need to be trained in this area. No one will want to hire a fitness coach who does not have the necessary certifications. The earning potential will depend on the type of clients you deal with and the exact services you offer.

9. **Training-Center Business with Continuing Education—** Maybe you have a passion for passing on your skills to others so they can make a difference in people's lives with respect to their health. If so, this business may be for you. It involves opening a training practice and teaching people to pass on your skills. You will need to have the expertise and appropriate qualifications in order to train people. Also, depending on how complex you would like your business to be, you may need to get special licenses. If you choose this business, don't be too forceful with your clients initially. Once people learn how to exercise their bodies and minds, they realize the importance of exercise and become willing to put in the hard work to exercise.

10. **Hosting Seminars and Workshops—**This option is for individuals with a physical space that they can use to host Health Care workshops and seminars. You will need to ensure that the premises are suitable for these types of events, and then you will rent that space to individuals and organizations.

11. **Health Care Informatics Consultant—**Health Care informatics involves the integration of information and communication technologies. Professionals in this field

seek to ensure the safe and efficient provision of Health Care services and the responsible creation and use of Health Care-related data, knowledge, and information. As a consultant, you will use your knowledge in computer science, information management, communication, epidemiology, cognitive science, management, and health science to guide Health Care professionals.

12. **Software Consultant**—There are numerous Health Care software programs available today. However, few Health Care professionals have been fully trained in the proper and efficient use of such programs and software. If you are skilled in a particular type of software, you can offer your services as a consultant. Your earning potential will depend on how well you know the software and on the levels of service you are willing to offer.

13. **Health Care Business Coaching**—The choice is vast, and you can make a success as you navigate your way and be passionate about what it is that you are doing. If you love social media, love helping people, and have a strong background in the Health Care industry, you can build a great business. Entrepreneurs today understand the importance of social media and how it can help them grow their business. One of the main problems they have, however, is that they either do not have the time to manage their social media themselves or they do not have the skills required to do so. Their solution is to get someone to manage this aspect of their business. The problem is that sometimes they hire people who are not knowledgeable about their industry, and this is why social-media management may be a great opportunity for you. As someone with a background in the Health Care

industry, you have an advantage in managing the social-media presence of businesses in the industry. There is a very low start-up cost here, low overhead, and the income potential is huge.

14. **Weight-loss Business**—A large percentage of the American population is becoming more concerned about their weight and is seeking opportunities to get in shape. The time is now to take advantage of the opportunities weight loss is offering. People are aware that they have a weight problem and are willing to take steps to correct it—especially women. They are concerned about their weight, but they do not consume enough dietary fiber to keep the body in shape. The beauty of a weight-loss business is that you can start it from home if you want to do so. Buying a weight-loss franchise is another, more expensive, option. In order to start your weight-loss business, however, you will need to be skilled in this area, trained, and possibly have a license—depending on where you plan to start your business. Your income will depend on your clientele and your level of skills and qualification.

15. **Stress-Management Coach for Health Care Professionals**—As a Health Care professional, you are aware of how stressful Health Care careers can be. You probably also know that it is just as important to take care of yourself as it is to take care of your patients so that you can continue to provide care for them as long as possible. This situation provides a wonderful opportunity for you to become a stress-management coach for your fellow Health Care professionals. Many Health Care providers seek services from their nearest hospital or psychiatric counselor to address issues with anxiety or depression. You can help them

by promoting a healthy and stress-free life—and you can benefit by getting some handsome fees. As a Health Care professional who understands the stress this career creates, you will already have some established credibility in the field. You need to be able to help people reduce stress and respond well to a range of different stressors. People will be more willing to use your service since they will be able to identify with you and you with them. You may need special training and certification depending on what state you are operating in. Your income potential will depend on your ability to launch such a business and the type of clients you will be serving.

16. **Executive Health Care Leader: Coach and Consultant—** If you are someone with many years of experience in the Health Care industry, then being a coach and consultant can provide you with a great business opportunity. Every day new people join the Health Care field, and some of these people—in an effort to do their best—may look for a mentor or coach who can help and guide them on their Health Care journey. You can offer your services to up-and-coming Health Care professionals. You will need to have experience, skills, and training in the areas they are trying to get into. Your income potential will depend on your ability to properly market your business as well as the amount and type of clients you will have. Not everyone may seek a coach or consultant when getting started in the Health Care industry, but those who are serious about their success will.

17. **NCLEX Training—**Many Health Care professions require some sort of examination before granting a license. One such license is the NCLEX (National

Council Licensure Examination). This provides a great opportunity for you to start a new business offering training and classes to help people prepare for the NCLEX in the same way that many schools and individuals provide training for examinations such as GMAT. NCLEX training can occur in many ways, depending on how individuals learn best. You will, of course, need to understand the exam. You will need to have passed the exam yourself and be able to help people prepare for it, and you must have served as a nurse prior to offering test-preparation services. The amount you can charge for this service will depend on how in-depth you plan to go with your training and classes. You may need a special license to offer classes depending on where you plan to do this, so check with the business bureau in your area.

18. **Cardiac Pulmonary Resuscitation/Automated External Defibrillation (CPR/AED/First-Aid) Training**—This option is similar to the previous business idea, as you would be offering training and classes. You would organize classes for CPR, AED, and first-aid training to provide help for people who are interested in renewing their certifications or who are studying for the first time. This type of training allows people to deal with injuries and medical emergencies that may occur at work, play, or elsewhere. This is a great business opportunity because many different individuals—not only Health Care professionals—seek training in these areas, especially first aid. There are many organizations that may offer this type of training, such as the Red Cross. However, being able to package your service in a unique way and putting your personal touch on your classes will allow you to enter the market

easily. You will need to be trained and have certification in these areas to be able to do this type of business. Your income potential will depend on how much you decide to charge for your services and who you are offering your services to. Once the training is complete, the participants will receive a certificate of completion. You can easily step up your charges as you earn further certification and degrees. This is a good business for attracting repeat customers. The certificates provided in these areas come with an expiration date, so the participants will likely be back in the future to maintain their certification status.

19. **Online Writing for Health Care Websites and Marketers**—There are many Health Care blogs and websites that are always looking for content. Depending on your expertise, you can write about specific Health Care topics for those in the market for this information. Individuals all over the web are continuously updating their websites or providing more sources of Health Care information for their targeted audiences. Furthermore, this could be a chance to inform audiences about your particular ideas and learning gleaned from the Health Care industry. Many of these people are willing to pay for content written for their audiences. You can charge per word or per project depending on your preference and the agreement with your client. You need to be able to write well and have something of value to say that will inspire, entertain, and educate.

20. **Adult Day-Care Center**—These types of centers are designed to help senior citizens who are no longer able to operate independently or those who are lonely or isolated. Seniors are able to socialize with each other while

receiving much-needed care. Many of the senior citizens in the United States feel helpless. They think they did enough for their country and its people, but they are getting nothing in return. You can open you own adult day-care center, and it can be private, public, or even a nonprofit. This type of business venture is for you if you have a passion for getting elders out of their houses to receive mental and social stimulation. In many cases, the senior citizens' caregivers are those who will pay for your services, in order to free them up to attend to their own needs.

21. **Child Day-Care Services**—This service is similar to the previous business opportunity. If you are interested in offering day-care services—but not for adults—you could offer this service to children. Running a day care will involve having a place that can accommodate children on a daily basis so that parents with young kids can continue to work or attend to personal needs without worrying about their children's care. If you want to take autistic or otherwise disabled children, you will need the proper education and experience. You may not be required to have special certification. However, you must be able to deal with kids and have a space that is welcoming to children. Having training in this field will be an added benefit to your business. Your income potential will depend on the rates you set for parents to pay for this service.

22. **Ghostwriting for the Medical Profession**—There are numerous authors out there looking for people with expertise in the medical field to write for them. If you have experience and expertise in the medical field, you can work as a ghostwriter, writing books and reports on

behalf of someone else. You will need to thoroughly understand the topic the person is asking you to write about, and you will also need excellent writing skills and a command of the language the book or report is written in. The income potential here will depend on how well you can write, your level of expertise, and also how you charge. You can charge per project, or you can charge per word. There are many freelance websites, such as freelancer.com, where you can offer your services. I remember when I was writing my first book and became stuck that the first thing that came to my mind was, "Are there any Health Care professionals who are ghostwriters?" I am still not sure if there are that many around. If you decide to launch a business in this area, not only are you creating more information to change lives, but you are opening up opportunities for more books to be produced.

23. **Medical Inventor**—The Health Care industry is always open to new ideas. A medical inventor can introduce new ideas in the medical field based on expertise as a Health Care professional. Nurses and other Health Care professionals who deal with clients on a daily basis tend to see ways to improve the system and make jobs easier. If you have an idea for something that can be invented to help improve the industry, then this could be the start of a health business. Or, you might be able to sell your idea to another company, which could result in royalties for you in the form of monetary payment and other forms of compensation.

24. **Companion-Care Business**—Companion-care businesses usually do not offer medical care to people but provide

services such as supervision, cooking, cleaning, and transportation, mainly in clients' homes. Although one does not necessarily have to come from the medical industry to open such a business, having a medical background will help the business succeed since the caregivers will be able to give better care to clients. The income potential will depend on the type of clients that you acquire. This can be a very lucrative venture that provides an excellent return on your investment.

25. **Private-Duty Care**—This opportunity involves providing personal, one-on-one care to people who can afford to pay for such services. Some people would rather have private-duty care because of the one-on-one attention and the continuity of having the same provider take care of them. These services are normally exclusive and very costly; however, there are people willing to pay for personalized care. Your income potential will depend on your ability to find the right client who will be willing to pay the required cost of the service. When marketing yourself, emphasize your talents and experience.

26. **Staffing Agency**—One of the business activities that many entrepreneurs dislike—especially in the Health Care industry—is that of hiring and staffing. Helping these entrepreneurs staff their businesses will free up enough time for them to focus on other aspects of their venture. Here are some different types of staffing agencies to consider:
   - Temporary-staffing agency
   - Long-term-staffing agency
   - Temporary-to-long-term agency

In this business, you help recruit the best candidates for various positions that companies have available. As compensation, each company or facility will agree to a certain monetary percentage based on the number and experience of the staff that is provided for a given amount of time. One of the most popular specialties in this field is placing nurses in businesses, hospitals, and other organizations that need them.

27. **Health Care Author and Writer**—Blogging, article writing, and ghostwriting were previously mentioned. However, there is also the opportunity to write for yourself. If you have something to say and you believe people need to hear it and it will make a difference in their lives, then maybe writing a book is for you. In order to write a book, you need to have expertise in a particular area. No one will bother reading a medical book written by someone who has no affiliation to the medical field or isn't trained as a medical professional; good credentials are necessary to build credibility and loyalty. The income potential from writing is huge. Your income, though, will depend on the type of book you write, your level of expertise, and how well you market your book.

28. **Health Care Advocacy: Empowering Patients**—Health Care advocates organize support and educational services to help maintain, improve, and manage their clients' health. People in the Health Care industry—such as doctors and nurses, among others—are the ones who generally become Health Care advocates. This is a great business for you if you are interested in going above and beyond for patients and helping them manage their health. If you are interested in this field, you need to learn the laws where you live

concerning the Health Care advocacy industry. Patient advocacy is what all Health Care professionals should strive for, despite their own beliefs. The patient should always be the center of focus when providing care. Advocacy should always be encouraged and emphasized at all times in the Health Care industry. Having patients who are empowered will result in more positive care outcomes. When patients are involved in the decisions made related to their health, they will feel that their wishes are being carried out as well as possible. Income potential here will vary depending on how you set up your business; many Health Care-advocate services are social enterprises and nonprofits.

29. **Affordable Care Act and Health Care-Reform Training—** The Affordable Care Act will affect employers in major ways until it is fully implemented in 2018, and beyond. It is important to provide training and information to employers so that they can understand all requirements and changes. The execution of this business idea is similar to the one above, and the income potential will vary depending on how the business is set up. Many agencies are offering this information for free. However, even with free content, there are different ways to monetize the information or receive special grants to execute the business.

30. **Critical-Care and Emergency-Services Training—** Unfortunately, accidents happen frequently. This provides a great opportunity for Health Care professionals to organize a business to provide individuals with the training and knowledge they need in order to be equipped to handle emergency situations. These types of training are specialized, and you will need to be qualified and properly

trained. Depending on your state, there may be special requirements. You will need to check with your local business bureau as well as the Health Care secretariat. Your income potential will depend on your fee scale as well as your ability to sell your services to others. Check with other businesses in your state to figure out how much they are charging, and price your services accordingly.

31. **Continuing Education**—This is a great business for people interested in teaching and in helping Health Care professionals continue their education; however, this business is not very easy to start with a small investment. Providing continuing education is especially ideal for people with extensive experience and education. There are many nurses and other Health Care professionals who want to continue training in order to improve their skills, and providing an avenue for this can be very beneficial to you. Depending on your state, you may need a special license to start this type of continuing-training school. Your income potential will depend on how much you decide to charge for your services, minus your overhead costs.

32. **Certified Health Care-Assistant Training Center**—This business is similar to the preceding opportunity; however, the focus here is to establish a training center to train Health Care assistants. You will be supplying or providing training to individuals who express interest in becoming effective Health Care assistants. You may choose to participate as an instructor in such a program. If you have years of experience, you may even feel that it is your duty to teach others. Take a look at the other training centers in your area to get an idea of how to price your services.

In order to do this business, you will need to have the proper training and certifications as well as industry experience and expertise that you can pass along to trainees. Launching a Certified Nursing Assistant school is one of the most lucrative business ventures that a Health Care professional could pursue. This is one of those businesses where you are constantly touching lives and making a difference every day. Training individuals to assist the needy is very rewarding and, whether you choose to be the trainer or the owner, understand that you are indeed changing lives. Patients are the most important element in the entire Health Care arena. They need your help and the help of others.

33. **Health Care Informatics and Computer Maintenance—** Idea number 11 describes the option of becoming a Health Care informatics consultant (using your knowledge in computer science, information management, communication, epidemiology, cognitive science, management, and health science to guide Health Care professionals). The opportunity presented here, however, involves maintaining the systems used in the Health Care industry. If you have been working with the technologies and special computers used for providing Health Care services, then you have a great opportunity to offer your services as a freelancer or registered business to maintain these computer systems. You will need to provide certifications and credentials showing that you are able to do the required tasks; however, the revenue potential here is huge.

34. **Home-Health Agency—**There are people who require special medical treatment and prefer to have the

treatment at home. These people may require a specialized form of care that only a medical expert can provide. This provides an opportunity for you, as a Health Care professional, to offer services to these people. You will need to have a specialty in a particular area that people will be willing to pay for. In this type of business, you need to have strong marketing to convince people how important the program is. You will need to have your license, and it must be up to date. (This also applies to anyone you will have working with you.) Your income potential will depend on the number of clients you can attract. One of the best ways to market this type of business is by word of mouth, based on a great reputation.

35. **Assisted-Living Facility**—These are retirement communities designed for people needing on-site assistance with things like personal care, medication, and mobility. The residents may be old or young, but they will all need some kind of assistance with activities such as cooking, mobility, bathing, housekeeping, eating, and getting around. If this is something you are interested in, then it is a great opportunity for starting a business. You need to be genuinely interested and passionate about helping people. The revenue potential is huge, but it will depend on how well you can market your services.

36. **Health Care School**—This opportunity is for people who want to start a school to train Health Care professionals. Such a business would be challenging to set up; however, starting a school is a great opportunity to help train the next generation of Health Care professionals. You will need certain permits, adequate facilities, and the

qualifications to teach. If you are not qualified to teach, you will need to hire instructors. The income potential from your school will depend on your ability to attract students who will want to train with you.

37. **Nursing Home**—Many people will prefer to live in their home as they get older. But, in many cases, there just isn't anyone at home to take care of them. This type of business gives you a chance to create that home away from home. You will need to have people on staff who are medically trained and able to take care of these people. In many cases, these types of organizations are nonprofit and charitable organizations and all require special licenses to operate. Specific regulations will depend on your state. Your income potential will depend on the number of people in your care and the amount you are charging to take care of them.

38. **Health Care Retail Business**—This kind of business involves purchasing and selling Health Care products and is a great opportunity for many individuals. There are many companies promoting health products to customers through a retailer, and you can be one of them. This is a relatively easy business to start since there may not be special medical licenses required on your part; however, you may need to have a license to sell certain medical products, especially if they need to be recommended by a doctor. People are becoming more aware of their health and are always looking for healthy products. The success of this business depends a lot on your ability to run a retail business. There are many business-management courses available that you can take to build your skills as an entrepreneur. This training is important because it will determine your income potential.

**39. First-Aid Kit Business**—Different countries have different health-and-safety regulations that govern workplaces. In some places, one regulation is that every employer should have a first-aid kit on site in case of employee sickness or injury. This provides a great business opportunity for you to create and sell first-aid kits to these businesses or to anyone needing one. You do not have to make the items in the kit yourself; you will simply put the kit together. This kind of business is relatively easy to start. You just need to form a small company and find some cheap labor. The business potential here is huge, and the income potential will depend on how well you can sell your first-aid kits.

**40. Medical-Software Programs Business**—This business is not only for people in the Health Care industry but for anyone in the software-development industry with a background in Health Care. With the increase in technology and reliance on electronic medical records, one of the biggest business opportunities out there today is that of creating software to support the efficient delivery of Health Care. Even if you have no software-development experience, if you have an idea, you may be able to team up with someone who has the necessary knowledge to create the software.

**41. Alternative Health Care Center (Aromatics-Herbal Treatment)**—This business involves moving away from the idea of conventional medical care to provide herbal or plant products as a cure for those who are sick. Many of these highly concentrated, fragrant oils—rich in chemical compounds—are extracted by steam distillation from flowers, leaves, roots, seeds, and bark and used in aromatherapy. It is important to note that not all leaves and herbs are safe for use. However, individuals are seeking this type of treatment more and more, allowing Health Care professionals to generate income as entrepreneurs in this sector.

42. **Doula Services (Help Laboring Mothers)**—If you are good at and interested in providing physical and emotional support to women during childbirth and the early-postpartum period, then this is a great opportunity for you. I think it is the most profitable business in the Health Care field. Most women become pregnant at some point, and they need nursing during pregnancy and at the time of delivery. If you have expertise in clinical practice, this will be the highest paying and most valuable job. You will improve women's pregnancy-and-labor experience by offering continuing information and working as an advocate for your client. This is a great business opportunity, and your experience in the Health Care industry will make it relatively easy to enter. The income potential is great as there are plenty of women seeking extra support during their pregnancy.

43. **Natural Childbirth Class**—Lots of women and couples are looking for ways to prepare for birth and labor. This presents a great opportunity to offer classes that cover topics such as signs of labor, normal progress of labor and birth, and techniques for coping with pain. If you are able to offer classes in this areas, then this business is for you. You can also team up with birthing centers and midwives to offer your service to their clients.

**44. Online Medical-Information Resource Center**—This is an online business where people can connect to a website to get information about a sickness they are facing or about medical practitioners in their area. This type of site will allow people to ask questions and get feedback from a medical professional like you. This business opportunity is for you if you have a passion for sharing information with people who need it. Many of the physicians in Western Europe and the United States are prescribing medications to patients through online portals to reduce patient fees. There are different ways that a website or online portal can be monetized, from charging a monthly listing fee to medical practitioners to selling advertising spots and informational products.

**45. Launching Community Health Fairs**—if you are interested in event planning as a Health Care practitioner, then this opportunity is for you. This business involves organizing health fairs where people can participate in health talks and have opportunities to buy important health products. Activities at health fairs involve things like complimentary lab work, blood-pressure reading, and blood-glucose checks. Those free tests serve as an incentive for individuals to come out and participate. Hundreds of medical schools in the United States launch this type of fair in their area and get useful results. Organizing these types of activities can be a significant source of income for the organizer. You can charge a fee for attending some of the talks and conferences at the fair. Also, the sale of healthy products can provide revenue for you. Other people may request to participate in your fair to sell their Health Care products or offer their services; these people can be charged a small fee for attending the events and offering their services.

46. **Medical-Braces Business**—This is another great opportunity for Health Care professionals. You can start providing medical braces to people who need them. The great thing about this business, like many others, is that you do not have to make the braces yourself. You do need to find a reputable supplier that can provide exactly what you need at a cost that will allow you to make a profit when you sell.

47. **Medical-Equipment Sales**—You might have medical equipment and other medical supplies that you are not using and can offer for sale—things like glucometers, insulin pens, blood-pressure monitors, and stethoscopes. You may also be able to procure some of these types of equipment and supplies from people who are willing to sell them to you. Then you, in turn, could offer them to a final consumer. This is a great opportunity, and the income potential will depend on your ability to sell to others.

48. **Mobile Hearing Testing**—This business involves providing hearing-testing services for people in various locations and managing the data from such testing so as to help people improve and maintain their hearing quality. Many people have problems with their hearing and will welcome this service—especially since it is mobile and will go to them, as opposed to them coming to you.

49. **Vitamin Sales**—Another great business opportunity is that of selling vitamins to people who need them. While this may be similar to other retail businesses, having a business that exclusively focuses on selling vitamins is a good opportunity because people tend to go to specialist

shops to get certain products. Branding yourself as an entrepreneur whose business is exclusively vitamins will appeal to many people, and the income potential from this is huge.

50. **Home-Care Education for Quality Measures in Hospitals**—As a Health Care professional, you can educate people about the right way to take care of themselves at home to avoid certain illnesses. Educating people about matters such as personal hygiene can really help them in the long run. It is surprising how many people are unaware of how to take care of themselves. This opportunity is for you if you have a passion for people and for helping them. The income potential in this business depends on your ability to sell your services to people. Depending on how you decide to impart this education, you may require a teaching license.

# CHAPTER 4

## THE HEALTH CARE CLIMATE

The Health Care industry can be intimidating, challenging, yet rewarding—all at the same time. Health Care is one of the most compelling, complicated, and rapidly growing industries in the country and throughout the world. Those who choose to delve into this special climate should be prepared for challenges at any point. If you enter the Health Care industry as an entrepreneur, you should ensure that you possess a strong knowledge base, and always be ready to back up your thoughts with logical reasoning. This will help you establish yourself in a leadership position that will eventually take you to the top. Health Care is the supreme profession of all professions in the world. To be successful you need to be level-headed, helpful, kind to others, well-mannered, professional appearing, and strongly dedicated. Always remember that you are the last one in the world before God.

The Health Care industry will continue to change and grow, and not just through government intervention. More and more, Health Care is being taught as a way of life, rather than as a crisis one has to deal with. Annual doctor visits are on the rise, and more employers are supporting healthy lifestyles through incentive programs—such as reimbursement for gym member-ships and employee-education initiatives.

With President Barack Obama's new Health Care law, there is a real possibility for expansion of Health Care coverage. The hope is that this expansion will encourage those Americans who are newly insured to seek out needed elective medical care that they may have been putting off. Another hope is that, with the expansion of coverage, the levels of uncompensated care will decrease.

Other proposals that have been put into action include those that are related to meaningful use within the Health Care indus-try. "Meaningful use" refers to the process of using certified elec-tronic-health-record (EHR) technology to improve the safety of care, ensure better quality of care, and ensure that the Health Care provided is as efficient as possible, while at the same time reducing Health Care incongruity. The process of meaningful use is comprised of three stages. The implementation of mean-ingful use will affect the Health Care climate because hospitals and providers will have difficult challenges as they strive to reach the bar that has been raised to meet the requirements of stage two and stage three of the process.

The Health Care climate is ever changing, with new advanc-es made more quickly, it seems, as time goes on. The economy seems to be the foremost challenge of the Health Care climate presently. The tight economy poses obstacles for funding medi-cal education, clinical care, and research. The negative impact that the economy is having on research has come at a time when research has already done so much for the industry but could do so much more. It's difficult to see medical-research support de-cline when there have been so many positive outcomes, leading to improved health in the general population.

Another challenge in the Health Care climate is the fact that we are being pushed to control Health Care costs. In some areas we are reducing costs rather dramatically, while also striving to improve quality, safety, and access for patients. Generally, a decreased demand for Health Care will reflect a decrease in costs, generating a positive effect on the economy. Preventive care is being greatly encouraged at this time. If a large majority of the population were to participate in preventive-care services, these services could improve their health and well-being for the future, resulting in fewer chronic diseases and decreasing the amount of money spent on treating those chronic illnesses.

Health insurance is also a huge issue in today's society. Some Health Care providers have been known to adjust their practices depending upon whether their patients have health insurance, but we should do our best not to attach a stigma to our patients who do not have insurance. On the other hand, health insurance has become more accessible for many, with hundreds of health-insurance companies providing multiple options.

As for professionals in the current Health Care climate, many career paths are potentially very rewarding. However, as with every other profession, it is not perfect, and there will be bumps along the way. When you chose to become a professional in the Health Care industry, you signed up for long hours, a lifetime of education, daily challenges, situations that push your boundaries, the need to manage rebukes for misunderstandings or mistakes, and many other hurdles that may make you second-guess yourself and what you signed up for. As an entrepreneur in the Health Care field, such issues will continue to be extremely overwhelming. You must embrace the difficulties from the very beginning and never fail to step up to face all challenges that are thrown at you. With the experiences you begin to have starting from day one, you will grow daily and will eventually become a leader that everyone else will look up to.

Flexibility is a characteristic that one must always be able to fall back on in the Health Care business. You will see that change occurs frequently, sometimes even on a daily basis, and you must be prepared to accept these changes, implement new ways to adapt, and move forward. Ultimately, if you can do that as an entrepreneur, your endeavor will provide you with great success.

# CHAPTER 5

## BUSINESS OWNERSHIP

T he journey of owning your own business will take you to both the mountains and the valleys at one point or another. The freedom of being your own boss and of being in control of your own destiny does indeed bring with it a sense of elation. However, you should expect to have to sacrifice a certain amount of that freedom in the beginning to get the business on its feet. Normally, everyone who builds a new business has to sacrifice time with loved ones. The sacrifices will be at the beginning of the process, and the joy comes farther down the road when you reach a level of maturity and decide it is time to hand over the reins and let someone else run the business for you. You—as well as the team you put together—will have invested loads of hard work and commitment before your company is mature enough for you to allow someone else to take over.

You have now made the decision to put your energy into making your own dreams a reality instead of working toward someone else's. Owning a business within the Health Care industry can prove to be a complex journey. The responsibilities are vast and come with both advantages and disadvantages. You will end up performing many different roles in your business that you might never have thought of. Running a business can be very taxing on your daily life, requiring you to put in many long days and to be available 24/7, especially in the beginning. Usually, when you decide to start a business, you either know exactly what you want to do, or you do not really have any definite ideas about how you are going to go about it. Those with a strong sense of what they are looking for in their business usually have already developed many of the skills necessary for success, and they are simply waiting for an opportunity to knock at their door and for the resources to jump-start their business.

The task of business ownership tends to be a bit less difficult for those who know exactly what they want out of their business. Whether you have a clear plan or not, you must be willing to work hard all the time, be persistent, keep up-to-date with your skills, have a strong sense of perseverance—and maybe even a little luck—to become successful and stay that way. If you really want to establish yourself as an owner, you must know what makes others successful in your prospective field and follow them. The more you prepare yourself for your endeavor, the more success you will have.

You also must come to realize that what you decide to do will almost certainly not be entirely unique. It is extremely likely that there are many other people in the world who also do what you want to do—so *what* you do is not the magical part of your business. The magic will stem from *why* you do it, *whom* you do it for, and *how* you do it. Once you discover your who, what, why, and how combination, you will be literally in business. A successful entrepreneur will always listen to everyone, especially consumers. You must always remain professional and stick to your values, even if you do not totally agree with what someone else believes. You can let the consumers always think they are right; just keep in mind that you will not be able to please everyone. However, you will quickly realize that your consumers are the most important assets in your business because who else is helping to pay your bills?

There is only one of you, so you must realize that you cannot do everything. Swallow some pride, and allow others to assume some roles within your business. Hire wisely, and invest in training for your staff in order to instill your business values and goals. You need to make sure that the individuals you hire fulfill their positions on your team and act in your business's best interests. Also, be sure that you can trust them to always be passionate about excelling in their positions. I have always relied on the phrase, "Work smarter, not harder." You will be in control of who holds positions in your business, so if at any time you feel someone is not working out, you can decide who to let go and when to do it.

To set yourself apart from other business owners, you need to think like your consumers. In this way, you will be able to anticipate their needs and meet those needs in innovative ways. Being able to do this is a key to success, because your consumers will know that they will be able to count on you to meet their needs better than anyone else can.

# CHAPTER 6

## YOUR *WHY* AND YOUR *PASSION*

I f you decide that you want to pursue your dreams and become an entrepreneur, then obviously you have a great
amount of passion that has steered you in this direction. You
should never hesitate when someone asks, "Why did you choose
this as your career?"

There has probably been someone in your life—a family
member, a friend, a coach, a coworker, or a teacher—who has
made a difference in your life and is part of why you are where
you are today. This person may have influenced you when you
were young, just recently, or both. You may have been influenced
by a positive experience, or it may have been the total opposite.
Either way, you have grown from that experience and that person, and this has come to be your *why* for what you have become
passionate about.

Most children have to face situations where others would like
to influence their career choice: Papa wants me to be a doctor.
Mama wants me to be an engineer. Grandpapa wants me to be
a lawyer. But ask *yourself* why you are making this career choice.
You're *why* is the most important thing you can figure out right
now at this point in your life. It is the reason behind the things
you are passionate about. If you do not know your *why*, you

will never be able to fully reach your personal and professional dreams. You must come to know yourself before you can provide for others.

The successful person should always be able to answer this question: "What is the passion that makes you excited to jump out of bed early each morning and take on the world?" Choosing to become an entrepreneur takes a special person who has strong values, traits, and characteristics. You must ask yourself, "Why would this career path make me want to jump out of bed each morning and take on the world?" If you are unable to tell someone why you have chosen such a position, you probably are not fully aware of your own beliefs and should work on clarifying them before you take on the responsibility of becoming an entrepreneur. You must be 100 percent aware of yourself and what you want out of life before you can share it with others or even think about becoming successful. The toll of being a Health Care entrepreneur will be extreme; you will push yourself to your limits on a daily basis. Whether or not you will be able to maintain perspective and continue to make a positive impact as you move forward in your success will depend on the amount of passion you have in the beginning. If you are passionate about something in your life, there is nothing that should be able to interfere with your success. If you ever find yourself struggling or second-guessing your decision, take time to step back and view the big picture and analyze your situation—you've got this!

If you are truly passionate about your work and are giving 110 percent daily, you will have the greatest chance of achieving financial success. Having passion for what we do gives us more energy and increases our ability to work hard. We also tend to be more creative, search more persistently for solutions when difficult problems surface, and always strive to inspire others who work with us so that the environment beams with positivity.

Each of these elements helps to increase our chances of success. Ultimately, we tend to be the happiest when we are pursuing our passions in life, and that is the best kind of success we will ever achieve.

# CHAPTER 7

## FIFTY BUSINESS IDEAS IN THE BANK

Earlier in this book, you read about fifty different routes you can take to become self-employed as an entrepreneur in the Health Care industry. Now, after you have determined your *why* and your *passion*, you can decide which avenue of the Health Care industry you would like to pursue in order to grow a successful business. One of the fifty ideas just might serve to be the spark that lights the fire to start your exciting career.

Each of the fifty ideas comes with its own advantages and disadvantages and deals with different aspects of the Health Care industry. The opportunities are endless, and each one comes with the potential for great success. Your skills and interests will determine which pathway you will end up choosing and how much effort you will need to put into your venture to be successful.

# CHAPTER 8

## The Benefits of Owning a Health Care Business

A t no time should a business owner focus completely on financial gain, rather than on how to improve lives and make a difference. One becomes a business owner to *be more*, *have more*, and *give more*. By doing these things, you have the ability and opportunity to amplify your impact and your income.

Becoming the owner of any business is a huge decision that can prove to be overwhelming and rewarding at the same time. Owning a Health Care business can be beneficial to you in many ways and will provide you with a lifelong investment that will continually reflect your passion. Owning your business means that it can be what you want it to be and not what you have been trying to do to meet someone else's expectations. Your business can reflect your passion 100 percent, each and every day. The following reasons explain why making the choice to start your own business can be your best choice yet.

- **You are in control of your destiny.** Being in an entrepreneurial position will allow you to call the shots and make every decision crucial to the failure or success of your business. You can write your own future with your own hand. Nobody else will get in your way and cloud your vision. This doesn't mean, however, that there won't be obstacles in your way. You will have problems; however, you get to determine what is done in your business to resolve those problems.

- **You become a part of a family.** The culture of entrepreneurs is like a big family. A fellow entrepreneur will always be there to share knowledge and advice. Successful entrepreneurs have mentors they can look up to. You can find a mentor—someone who has done what you are planning to do—and let that person guide you as you build your empire.

- **You can change lives.** With what your business is going to offer, you have the opportunity to provide others with services that could have a huge impact on their lives. Changing the life of someone for the better is extremely rewarding. Your business should always be about making a positive difference in people's lives; once you do that, money will follow.

- **You will serve as a role model.** The success you achieve will serve as motivation and inspiration for the many people who look up to you. Remember, the Health Care industry is the best industry, and the employees working in it are some of the best human beings on earth, so become a role model for them. After you gain experience, you can also mentor up-and-coming entrepreneurs and help them achieve their dreams.

- **There will never be boredom.** Each day will present new challenges and a to-do list that is two miles long. You will be kept on your toes, and you will never lose your spark. Just view each day as another rung on the ladder that leads to the top—you can do this!

- **It's your business, your decisions.** Each and every decision that is made regarding your business is your responsibility; you are in total control. Whether the business succeeds or fails, you are responsible.
- **Find satisfaction.** Being a business owner takes a ton of hard work and dedication, but to be able to say, "Yeah, that's my company," with confidence is a euphoric feeling.
- **Never feel belittled.** If at any point in your career as an entrepreneur you feel that you have a new idea to incorporate in your business, you can put it into place right away. Since you are the boss, you do not have to wait for someone in a higher position to listen to your idea and put it into place for you.
- **It is all your creation.** The decision you have made to start your own business is all yours, so you can build it from the dirt to the sky, as big as you want.
- **You are your own boss.** Being your own boss allows for more time spent with your loved ones. This is generally something everyone wants in life, and becoming an entrepreneur makes family time much more of a possibility. It's your company and your schedule.
- **Work hard, play hard.** You get what you put into life. If you work hard day in and day out, you will subsequently reap the benefits. The harder you work, the more opportunities you will have.
- **Have the ability to give back.** Being a successful business owner will allow you to give back by contributing to charities and participating in charitable events. The feeling of being able to give back and support your local community is wonderful.
- **Maintain your health.** With the ability to create your own schedule, you can arrange your work in ways that benefit your own health. For example, you may wish to develop

a daily fitness routine. Because, let's face it, Health Care business owners should definitely look like they take care of themselves. You shouldn't work so hard that your health suffers.

- **Contribute to society.** Introducing your business and the services you offer to the general population may directly impact their lives.

- **No more punching the time clock eight to four.** You will find that time-management skills are your friend. Know that—despite the fact that you may not be caring for a patient from the bedside—you are still touching lives and making a huge difference in the lives of patients and others. Your work days can either be too long, too short, or just right. Make your goal "just right," and also try to reach the goal that your day is done only when your to-do list and all of your other responsibilities are taken care of for that day.

- **It's a colossal challenge.** Being the leader of a business and directing others to remain on the path to success is not easy. The struggles you experience will be life-changing, and you would never have obtained the knowledge you gain from them otherwise.

- **There's never a dull moment.** Becoming a business owner is definitely not a dead-end job. The tasks will change almost daily, and you will have many different roles throughout your career. Do not worry about losing interest; that's the last thing you'll do.

- **You can adapt.** If for some reason your business slows down and does not experience growth for a while, as a leader you can figure out ways to adapt. You will determine where changes should be made in order to get your business back up to speed or pass your competitors again.

- **Great minds think alike.** One result of becoming an entrepreneur is that you will meet many extremely intelligent individuals with the same inspirations as you. Keep those people on your good side because you never know when you may need a little advice.
- **The sky's the limit.** Owning your own business provides you with an endless medium for growth. There are no limits except those set by your energy level and schedule.
- **Do what you love, and love what you do.** What could be better than waking up every day to do a job that you absolutely love? There is no better feeling than being successful and loving the way you are doing it at the same time. Most people dread hearing the alarm clock go off every morning.
- **You will be appreciated.** Creating a successful business will require others to purchase your services and evaluate them. Hopefully, they think enough of your services to share their recommendation with others so that your clientele rapidly grows. Seeing that others review your services positively and that what you do impacts lives for the better will give you a sense of appreciation.
- **Enjoy lifelong learning.** You will always learn lessons—sometimes the hard way—in this world. There is no way to skip learning. However, the type of education that an entrepreneur gets cannot be taught in a lecture hall.
- **Have no fear.** You are in charge, so you can rest assured that if your company has to make cuts due to finances or a decrease in demand, you will never be the one let go.
- **No matter what, there is always someone worse off.** A bad day as an entrepreneur will beat a bad day working for someone else by a long shot. Even if the day is bad, take a step back and consider: you are still the boss. If

anyone was going to reprimand you, it would have to be a superior, and there isn't one.

- **There is no particular educational degree required.** You do not have to have the highest level of education possible to start a business. Anyone can become an entrepreneur, and the possibilities are endless. This doesn't mean education is not important—it is. However, you do not need an MBA or other advanced degrees to start your business.
- **Make it enjoyable.** If what you are doing seems boring, you have nobody to blame but yourself. Find ways to make the work environment fun, and everyone will be more productive and enjoy coming to work for you.
- **Provide for others.** As a business owner, you will be providing for other people. Your employees will count on your leadership and ability to make good decisions, as what you do could impact whether or not they get paid the next week. Always try to pay your employees on time; it is your duty.
- **That was then, this is now.** After you have run your business for a while, you should take some time to look back to see how much you have grown as a person. Personal success and growth of a business come hand in hand. The more you grow, the more your business will grow.
- **Problem? That's no problem.** After many bouts of difficulties and lessons learned, you will have discovered many new ways to solve whatever challenge is thrown at you.
- **The bigger they are, the harder they fall.** Throughout the creation of your own Health Care business, there will be times when you feel as if you have been knocked down and have hit rock bottom. It will be at these times when

you will gain wisdom and inner strength. As a result, you will learn to roll with the punches, get up, and strive harder toward your aspirations next time.

- **Discover maximum rush.** When you decide to take the leap and become an entrepreneur, most likely you will put your lifestyle and finances on the line. You are willing to go all in because you so strongly believe in something. This will prove to be a huge adrenaline rush because of the unknowns.

- **Dream big.** Becoming an entrepreneur allows you to dream as big as you want to. If you can envision and believe, it will *happen* for you. Nobody is stopping you from becoming a success. Just as strenuous exercise makes an athlete perfect, you—as an entrepreneur—can achieve and enjoy a beautiful and secure life through hard work.

This is only a partial list; the benefits of owning a business can be endless. The experience that you will gain will be unlike any other. The rewards you reap will be well deserved, and nobody will control your destiny but yourself.

# CHAPTER 9

## The Abundant-Ten Model

The other name for this model is "The Multiple Streams of Income Model." This chapter will show you ways to increase your income and generate more business based on your skills, your gifts, and your talents as well as your passion.

You cannot expect your business to become an empire overnight. If you have that mentality, it is time to start realizing that it will take a significant amount of focus and hard work. Success comes with trial and error, along with implementation of various ideas that enable your business to prosper and remain competitive in the industry. There are many routes you can take that will lead you in the right direction. Having multiple streams of income means that your business will have more than just one way to generate revenue. The following ten ways will prove to be the most effective for the continued success of your business.

- **Seminars.** Seminars are gatherings of several individuals with the same passion who come together for the purpose of discussing specific topics related to their businesses. Participating in seminars can help you develop different approaches to issues pertaining to your business. These gatherings tend to be interactive to allow participants to engage in discussions about the specific topics related to their profession. Seminars are most often led by one or two presenters—but there could be more, depending on the expected size of the group. The presenters will ensure that the discussions stay on track so that an optimal amount of information is shared regarding the specific topics.

A seminar may have several purposes or just one. For example, a seminar may be for the purpose of education, such as a lecture, and the participants will discuss a certain academic subject with the goal of gaining better insight into the subject so that they are better prepared to teach others. Other forms of educational seminars may be held to teach the participants updated skills or knowledge so participants can provide those they are teaching with the most current information possible. An example of a topical type of seminar would be one that covers how to start a successful Health Care business. At such a seminar, participants could gain a tremendous amount of knowledge, including tips about how to maintain such a big investment. Attending topical seminars regularly as a Health Care entrepreneur will ensure that you have the most up-to-date information to provide your clients so that they are 100 percent satisfied in every aspect of the services that you provide.

Seminars can also be motivational, with the purpose of inspiring participants to become better people or to work smarter by implementing the skills they may have learned from attending the seminar. For instance, a business seminar with a financial theme could teach small-business owners how to create a sales pitch that will wow investors and generate the money needed to start the business.

Most generally, though, you will go to—or even host—seminars to network with businessmen and businesswomen with interests similar to yours. Attending seminars will provide you with opportunities to make valuable contacts who will help you move to the next level in your endeavor.

- **Workshops.** A workshop is similar to a seminar; however, there are evident differences. The main difference is that seminars lean more toward academia, and the environment is less hands-on than at workshops. Seminars are events that are mostly geared toward topics regarding education and usually feature one or more experts who can present their real-life experiences on the subject matter. On the other hand, workshops are generally less formal and will require more participation from those in attendance. The main goal of the workshop is for those participating to gain new skills during the event that they can implement right away—under the guidance of a professional. Workshops will most always have a smaller group of people in attendance due to the hands-on environment and the time it takes for the professional to effectively demonstrate and impart the skills before the end of the session. Workshops will most likely have a few different activities that participants can engage in that all stem from the topic of discussion.

  Communication in the workshops also tends to be more of a two-way street. The professional in charge will share his or her knowledge and then will be open to anything you have to say once you are going through the process of the hands-on activities. Everyone seems to do tasks a bit differently, and sometimes it helps to see different routes that can be taken to get to the same end result. A different approach may be simpler in your particular situation and may result in greater success for your business.

- **YouTube.** Using videos that reach targeted audiences can be an impressive business technique that can skyrocket revenues and increase the likelihood of viewers choosing your Health Care service. It seems like—no matter where you are—if you look around, four out of five people will be on their cell phones. YouTube has helped many people be successful. Producing a video for your business should be a must.

  The video should be as professional as possible and should give your targeted audiences a feel for exactly what will be provided to them should they choose your services. Being able to see who is behind the whole deal makes it easier for audiences to become attracted to what you have to offer. Not very many people are willing to spend significant amounts of money on something that they have only read about. People generally rely on being able to see pictures of the product or being able to watch an interactive video that will thoroughly describe the product or service.

  The video does not have to be very long; it should just be a quick and simple overview of your business so that your audience can become familiar with the standards and values you offer in order to determine whether or not your business is a good fit for them. It is always a good idea to do a little research before just throwing a video out there on the web. Search for similar work, and see how the ratings fall. Based on your research, you should be able to generate a video that will be viewed and shared throughout the Internet.

- **Blogging.** A successful blog is a frequently updated personal journal that can be found via the Internet. A blog can be extremely beneficial to your business. It can be a way to connect personally with your audience and with those for whom you are providing services. In your blog, you can share your thoughts and your passions. Your blog can be whatever you want it to be; it is your choice. Blogging should support your business. Whenever something happens that you feel would reflect positively and further engage your audience, do not hesitate to begin writing! With a successful and engaging blog, you will be able to reach hundreds—or even thousands—of people on a daily basis, and that will have a huge impact on your business.

As an entrepreneur, you should remain professional in all your blogs. Don't delve too much into your personal life, but maintain focus on your professional passion. Through your blog's comment section, you will gain insight into how others feel about your business, and you should always be open to ways to make your business better. When it comes to Health Care, communication is key...and generally, it is lacking. In order to be a successful entrepreneur, you should always make others feel included and listen to their thoughts and concerns. The respect you will gain will be tremendous. The more others like you, the more likely they are to share with others, and in this way your business will have an increased ability to flourish.

- **CD/DVD.** You can increase revenue by selling these products through your business as informational sources to further spread the word about your Health Care business.
- **Social Media.** Social media has had an overwhelming impact on the way the general population interacts. With things like Facebook, Twitter, and Instagram, people can interact and connect in more ways than have ever before

been imagined. Generally, when it comes to finding information related to health issues, you will find that people turn to the web. Information about your business can be shared much more easily and more quickly by taking advantage of the tools of social media. The use of social media can be a positive asset to a business because you can share your content with thousands of followers, but that is not the only benefit. You can also gain knowledge about your audience, which can help you cater to your customers through special campaigns and product offers. Social-media use also allows consumers to provide instant feedback to you. From the feedback, you can learn about and implement ideas to make your business better from your customers' point of view.

- **Brochures and Magazines.** Traditional reading material is another good way to get the word out about your business. You must make the material attractive and informative enough to keep your potential customers' attention. It may be reasonable to mail the material to your immediate community to spread the word about what your business has to offer. (Of course, you must set your budget so that you do not place too much emphasis on the direct mailing aspect of marketing.) It is important to have brochures in your business office for consumers to take when they visit in order to continue to spread the word.

- **Upselling.** Upselling is a sales technique where a seller persuades the customer to purchase more expensive items, upgrades, or other add-ons in an attempt to make a more profitable sale. An example of this would be a discounted car-wash purchase after a customer fills the car's tank with gas.

- **Membership Website.** When you offer a paid membership website, you will continue to maintain your regular income each month, plus you can build upon your consumer base. You will find that it is much easier to sell to individuals who are already your customers than to find new ones. People enjoy being a part of a community where they can share their own thoughts and opinions, so joining a members-only website will be appealing to them.

- **Video Marketing.** Video marketing is an area that is quickly growing in the business industry. We are in the age of information overload. Therefore, it is crucial for businesses that are just starting out or continuing their growth to offer content that potential consumers quickly digest, or they will just move on to the next offer. Make your video creative, but ensure that it is direct and gets to the point so that you can grab the viewer's attention.

# CHAPTER 10

## HOW TO START

Beginning your own Health Care business is a huge decision that will most likely change your life forever; it is up to you to make sure your life is changed in a good way. There are several things to take into consideration when starting such a business. The following steps will help you ensure that you have a strong foundation upon which to build your business into a success.

- Research your market, and develop a network. Keep in mind that any new business venture requires a solid amount of research. Essentially, you are a little fish in a big pond. Your research will include evaluating the current market. Determine the number of businesses in your area that are similar to the one you plan to start, and evaluate their specialties and effectiveness. This will help you to determine if there is a need for the exact service you would like to offer, and you will be able to determine whether or not you need to create a diversified program to be competitive. Having a firm network of friends and colleagues is also a must. These people can help you spread the word about your business. You should surround yourself with those who support your thoughts and passion.

- Take a good hard look at yourself. What characteristics do you have that will help you to run a business? Are you sure you are ready to become an entrepreneur? You may have a strong passion for starting a business, but remember that you must be ready to give 110 percent at all times to guarantee your success—especially when beginning your business. You have to be prepared to get up early, work hard continuously, and stay up late. You must do this but also find time to take good care of yourself. Your good health is important because your business will not be able to function by itself. You will have to distinguish what sets you apart from all of the other people who may be offering something similar. The population looks for products and services that are new and cutting edge. You will not be successful by just blending in.

- Decide what kind of business you want, where you will operate your business, and who your target customers will be. Do you want a small instructional business, teaching skills such as CPR? Or is your passion to open a large home-health business to care for the aging population in their homes? The choice is yours. You will want to locate your business in a place that is growing and has the potential for long-term viability. Bear in mind, also, that you need to find a way to make what you do special so that no one else can easily copy your business model. You will also want to make sure that you have registered your idea because someone with more finances and a better marketing strategy can come along and copy your vision, turning it into his or her success.

After you research the market, determine what your driving force is and that you are ready to take the leap, and plan the details of your business, you are ready to go!

# CHAPTER 11

## MARKETING PLANS AND STRATEGIES THAT WORK

You generally need a business plan when starting a business. A formal plan is not always a must, but you must have some kind of a plan for where you are and where you are going in your business. However, some entrepreneurs forget that a marketing plan is just as crucial as a business plan. A marketing plan will be your strategy to win and keep customers. Your plan will highlight your customer-acquisition strategy and what you will need to do to keep those customers. A good marketing plan is a plan of action that details what you will sell, who will want to buy it, and how you will go about generating sales.

### Your Target Market

Before you can do anything else with your marketing plan, you need to know who your target market is. Target audiences have become highly specialized and segmented. No matter your industry, positioning your product or service competitively requires an understanding of what is going on in your target market. Not only do you need to be able to describe exactly who your market is, but you must also have a clear understanding of what your competitors are offering to be able to show how your product or service provides a better value. Think outside of the box when you consider your target audience, taking into account the values and passions your business is based on. Take time to sit down and make a list of the audiences your business is going to best target, and figure out the best ways to reach out to those segments.

## Unique Selling Proposition

In order to fully set yourself apart from your competition, you need to have a full understanding of your unique selling proposition. What is it that makes your business different from all the others? As a business owner, there are many factors you need to take into consideration to achieve success; however, it is important that amid all these things that you keep sight of the big picture—what makes you unique.

## Your Competitors

While your entire focus should not be on your competitors, you need to know what they are offering and how their product or service compares to your offerings. As you look at the total market for whichever Health Care business route you choose to take, you can better determine how much effort you will have to put into your marketing strategies. As was stated before, you must also develop your own unique selling proposition that sets you apart from everyone else. What can you offer a consumer that your competitors are not offering?

## Setting Goals

Setting goals within a reasonable time frame of around three to five years is another good idea. Decide where you want your business to be in the future, and decide what sort of marketing strategies will help you get there. Build a support team to help you reach your goals, and encourage enthusiasm. Associate with other experts in your area of specialty who will support your marketing efforts and help keep you accountable in meeting your goals.

## Pricing-and-Positioning Strategy

Your pricing-and-positioning strategy will send a message about your products or services. For instance, if you want to be known as premier and exclusive, having a very low price point will defeat this purpose.

## Distribution

You need to know exactly how you will go about selling and getting your products or service to your customers. Make a list of the ways that people will get your products, and refer often to it.

## Marketing Materials

Think about what types of materials are necessary as you begin your business. Needed materials to promote your business might include things like brochures and business cards.

## Promotion Strategy

This is one of the most important aspects of your marketing plan. Your promotion strategy will highlight how you will reach your customers; you can use television, radio, print, and online advertising. Online advertising has begun to overshadow the more traditional forms of advertising, and we will discuss this option in the next section.

## Online Marketing Strategies

Until a few years ago, online marketing was not a big part of most companies' marketing plans; however, today more and more companies are spending larger portions of their marketing budget on online marketing. One reason for this shift is that online marketing is now cheaper and more targeted than traditional forms of advertising. To be truly successful, your online marketing strategy needs to include the following:

- Social-Media Strategy—Use sites like Facebook, Twitter, LinkedIn, and Google+, among others, to engage and build a relationship with your customers and potential customers. Many small and large businesses are using social media to advertise, which we will discuss more fully in the next bullet point.
- Online Advertising—Facebook ads, Twitter ads, Google AdWords, and LinkedIn ads are some of the most common—and effective—forms of advertising used online. There ads are not as expensive as traditional forms of advertising, and they are more targeted and, therefore, more effective.
- Search Engine Optimization (SEO)—You need to ensure that your websites and other online assets rank well in online searches—whether through Google or Bing or another search engine. To achieve high rankings, you need to select keywords very carefully. Do not select too many common keywords that are widely used, since that may make it less likely that your company will appear high in the search rank.

## Joint Ventures and Partnerships

"No man is an island" is a famous quote from the English poet John Donne. This saying simply means that we all need someone in life. The same goes for business. You can team up with other entrepreneurs and businesses to conduct joint promotional strategies or host joint events, as well as form partnerships with these people. Joining forces can sometimes be the difference between a successful and a failed business.

There is a great African proverb that says, "If you want to go fast, go alone, but if you want to go far, go together." That is so true. It's amazing what we can accomplish when we make a decision to partner with other trusted entrepreneurs.

## Retention Strategy

There are many times when entrepreneurs go all out to build their clientele yet have no plan to keep these people around. It is much easier and less costly to sell to an already existing customer or client versus seeking a brand-new client. Have a plan to retain your current customers and to provide maximum value for these customers. This is the core of service excellence. As business owners we cannot overestimate the importance of taking care of our clients, our students, and our customers.

## Financial Projections

It is vital to document all the expenses you expect to have and that you employ only the strategies that will give you the highest return on investment. When in doubt, hire an accountant. Hire to compensate for your weaknesses, and capitalize on your areas of competence.

# CHAPTER 12

## GROWING YOUR BUSINESS

B usiness start-ups go through a life cycle just like living things. The early business life cycle includes choosing services or products, generating sales, and growing. Establishing a business is a huge deal, and preparing your business for expansion requires even more hard work.

When preparing to grow, you should take a look at what you currently offer and decide if there is anything worth reconsidering. Is what you are currently offering going to be enough to enable your business to keep growing, or do some aspects of your business need tweaking, based on the research you have done? For your business to sustain long-term growth, you must continually assess what sets it apart from competitors. You should ask yourself, "What is unique about my business compared to the competition that makes consumers *want* to do business with me?" You will often find that you have to recalibrate, recalculate, and resuscitate your business in order for it to increase its level of success and profitability.

### Marketing

As mentioned in the previous chapter, marketing is crucial to your business. It can also be used to grow your business and take it to the next level. I tell my nurse entrepreneurs that they must carve out two hours every day to market their business in order for them to generate income. Investment in marketing is a positive move toward business growth. As your sales increase, there will likely be a decrease in the productivity rate of your marketing. You can counteract this trend by working to make sales easier. Marketing strategies will be vitally important at this time for the growth of your business. Another aspect of entering the growth phase of your Health Care business is that your consumer focus should switch. You should begin to pay less attention to gaining new consumers and more attention to retaining and upselling to current consumers.

## Upselling

Upselling is a sales technique that, as an entrepreneur, you are probably already familiar with. As explained earlier, upselling occurs when you, the seller, induce the consumer to purchase items that are more expensive, purchase upgrades to the current product, or buy add-ons. These things result in more profitable sales. One of your business goals should be to maintain customers for life by providing the most up-to-date product or service that best fits their demands. By the growth phase, you have already found your business's target audience. At this point in the growing process, you should be able to define your ideal customer, and you should be able to track and understand the ideal customer's purchasing trends to keep your growth on the right track.

## Maintain Cohesion

Maintaining cohesion within your business should be another goal you strive for when your business reaches the growth phase.

This means that you should do all you can to ensure that every individual who is a part of your team is aware of what is going on at all times. This sort of unity is crucial for maintaining success, because everybody needs to stay on the same page for consistency. At this point in your business, you should be able to measure changes that occur. If you are unable to measure change, you cannot possibly know how effective your business is. Work to identify which areas within your business need to be changed in order to maintain success.

Never be afraid to look to your competition. Research similar businesses and see how they are growing. Do not let your pride keep you from asking for advice. Based on your analysis of businesses like yours, develop your own unique ways to apply what you have learned toward your own strategies for continued growth. Do not get left behind!

## Build on Strengths

At this point of growing your business, I am sure that you are aware of your various strengths and weaknesses. Work to focus on your strengths instead of improving on your weaknesses. Your strengths have gotten you this far, so restructure your business environment to feed off of your strengths, and continue to build upon them to watch your business grow. You should only have employees on your team who abide by your company's values and who are inspired by your company's products and services. Do your best to invest in motivated and talented people who have a knowledge base related to your business. In this way, you may be able to hire fewer employees but pay them a little more. If business slows, you will know who has the most dedication by seeing who decides to stick around if wages must decrease for a short time.

Following a specific business plan will help you achieve success. Do your best as an entrepreneur to coordinate your strategies for the growth of your business and your customers' satisfaction. This will keep your customers happy, and they will keep coming back for more.

## Use Social Media

As explained previously, social media provides a unique opportunity for you as an entrepreneur. You can enhance your customer service through sites like Facebook and Twitter. Social media allows you to engage with your customers and build a relationship with them. You can talk directly to your customers and get to know exactly how they feel about your products and services, as well as learning what areas they think might be improved.

## Segment Your Market

In order to fully maximize your sales and grow your business, it is wise to concentrate on the ideal customer that you have identified and to offer your products accordingly. Trying to sell your products to everybody will be a sure strategy for failure. It is wise to carve out a niche and offer your product to that segment.

## Partnership

As previously mentioned, engaging in a partnership with other entrepreneurs and businesses can prove beneficial to you when you are trying to grow your business. Many small businesses complain that they are unable to compete with larger companies since these businesses tend to have the advantage of being able to form partnerships with their suppliers and other businesses. However, there is nothing stopping small businesses from doing the same thing. You do not necessarily have to try to form partnerships with the large suppliers; however, other small businesses may be happy to collaborate, and this can help all the participating companies to grow.

# CHAPTER 13

## Implementing Social Media in Your Health Care Business

Throughout this book the importance of social media for business has been highlighted. That's because, as someone who will be starting your own Health Care business, you should be aware that social media can play a great part in the process. You can use different social-media platforms to fully launch your business as well as to build and amplify your presence and your message. Using social media is one of the best ways to go from unknown to well known; however, many people jump into using social media for their business without a plan or any kind of strategy in place. Though social media can be very effective in helping you build your Health Care business, if it is not done properly, you will be wasting your time.

### Social-Media Audit

The first thing you need to do when implementing social media in your business is to conduct an audit. An audit is usually thought of as being most useful to already-established businesses with a social-media presence. Established businesses will look at the platforms they use and will evaluate how they are using them and who is using them—the amount of fans or followers. But an audit also is important for you when you are just starting your business, simply because you need to know if anyone is using your business name on social media. For example, recently the owners of a business named Evergreen Store created a Facebook page. After creating the page—including the name Evergreen Store—they tried to get a personalized link that would look like this: facebook.com/ever-green store. This link had already been taken by someone else. So you need to look at these types of issues to ensure that your business name is available on the different platforms.

## Social-Media Objectives
There are many reasons to use social media, including brand awareness, lead generation, customer service, and sales. You need to figure out your objective in using social media before you start using it.

## Social-Media Strategy
A strong social-media strategy is what many people lack when they are implementing social media in their business. Many business owners get into social media without a proper strategy, and then they complain that it is not working for them. Don't be someone who makes that mistake. Your strategy should include the following:

1- Tools to manage your account—such as Hootsuite for scheduling
2- A content-and-editorial calendar to keep you on schedule as you create content and send it out
3- Goals you hope to accomplish by using your earned, owned, and paid media

## Content Plan

Businesses that are having the most success with social media are those that are operating like media companies. This means that they are creating and sharing valuable, informative, inspiring, and educational pieces of content with their fans in a genuine way—instead of trying only to sell to customers all the time. This type of sharing creates a strong relationship between you and your community. Readers will begin to trust you and see you as a go-to source for information—which is a huge advantage, especially in the Health Care industry. After you have built a strong relationship with your community and they are engaged and trust you, it becomes easier to sell those followers your products and services or other products and services that you may recommend.

## Advertising on Social Media

In the past, large companies have always had an advantage over smaller businesses because of the size of their advertising budgets. Larger companies were able to reach more people using traditional media platforms such as television, radio, and print media simply because they were able to pay for it. Smaller companies suffered and had no way to compete effectively with these larger companies. Social media has changed all that. Larger businesses no longer have an advantage over smaller ones because of the size of their budget; the playing field has been leveled. The reason is simply because social-media advertising is affordable for nearly everyone. Social media does have a few disadvantages. Nevertheless, it is certainly not as expensive as placing TV or radio advertising.

Platforms such as Facebook, Google, LinkedIn, and Twitter have all integrated advertising in their platform. Facebook, however, has one of the most robust advertising platforms, and it is also one of the cheapest. Anyone can create and run an ad, spending as little as five dollars a day, and have that ad shown only to a targeted group of people. Compare this to spending at least $400, or much more, for a one-minute spot on local television, where there is no guarantee that the people seeing the ad are interested in what you have to sell. With online advertising you can be sure that your ad will only be shown to the people you want to see it.

To create an ad on Facebook, you select your ad objective—whether you want to use website conversion or clicking to a website and page-post engagement among others—and follow the prompts to start creating your ad. Whether you are looking to produce leads, build brand awareness, get more fans, or sell a product, you can accomplish your goal using Facebook advertising, and you will not have to pay the huge amount you would pay to have an ad on TV. This is one of the best things about Facebook and other online advertising platforms.

In today's culture almost everyone is online and connected to some sort of social platforms. If you truly want to build and grow a successful business, you have to be where your customers and potential customers are. Remember, however, that social media will only work for you when it is done properly. Many people do not have the time or the technical knowledge to maneuver social media successfully, so they hire social-media management companies to help them. Whether you promote your business through social media yourself or hire an outside company to help you, social media can give you a decided advantage.

# CHAPTER 14

## ANOTHER LEVEL TO HEALTH CAREPRENEUR

The time to take your business to the next level has come—placing you face-to-face with the choices involved in making what was once your small business into something bigger. If you have been able to continually evaluate the vision and goals of your Health Care business, you should not be worried about taking the next leap. You have looked both on the inside and outside of your business: You have looked on the inside at your strengths and weaknesses, and you have looked on the outside at where you stand among other businesses in the Health Care industry. At this point, you should have great confidence in the strategies you are using for getting ahead and staying that way. In addition, you should be well aware by now of how you measure success within your business so that you will always know when the company is meeting your goals.

As a successful entrepreneur, you should always keep in mind your vision of where you want your business to be. If you always keep the end goal in sight and picture where you want to end up, you will continue to have the drive and motivation that you need to get there. Keep the journey exciting! You must maintain some level of excitement to enable you to keep climbing to the next level. In addition, always remember to take a little time to reward yourself and your team for all you have done up to this point and for what the future is going to hold for your business.

No matter what, keep climbing—even if you see that you have reached your business goal. That just means that it is time to set the next goal and keep on keeping on. Maintain an outstanding support system and solid teamwork. "Teamwork makes the dream work"—right? Ideally, your entire team should share your vision and understand the goals of your Health Care business in order to move forward smoothly. Every once in a while, take a break to look around. Take a little time to evaluate where you are, how you got there, and whether what you are doing is going to continue to help you reach your next goal on the next level.

Stick to your strengths, and build upon them instead of trying to tweak your weaknesses. You will find yourself taking one step forward and two steps back unless you focus solely on your strengths. Successful entrepreneurs will find themselves doing not only what they have to in order to get by, but they will go out of their way to do that much more. This will show your customers that you are always willing to go the extra mile for them. You will become the go-to person that they can always count on to get things done.

Keep your promises, and put an even greater focus on your consumers. If you continue to provide services for your regular customers, this will mean a continued regular income for you. Also, if you continue to keep your customers satisfied, you will be rewarded with the power of word-of-mouth recommendations to further boost your sales. Never shy away from asking consumers for their feedback, and act constructively when you receive this feedback. Address any concerns or issues brought to your attention quickly and thoroughly, while being consistently accountable for your actions. Being available to communicate with consumers is very important and will be a positive step toward your ultimate goals.

To maintain your position at a higher level of business, you must be able to commit yourself to lifelong learning and keeping up to date with technology. The Health Care industry is ever changing, with new ideas and technological advances emerging frequently. So, as an entrepreneur, you should always be adding to your knowledge so that you can adapt your services to remain competitive in this market. Plus, keeping up to date with the newest technology could save you time and money in the long run.

When your business is operating on a higher level, you should have your delegation skills almost perfected—whether you have employees, have subcontracted the work out, or just have family members helping you. Being able to delegate tasks can be the difference in reaching new levels or becoming burned out. As the owner of your business, you have played many roles and completed numerous tasks that require various skills. This may make it more difficult for you to delegate tasks. However, at this next level of growth, you will have learned what tasks you can delegate and to whom on your team. Then you can focus more on growing your business instead of being involved in the busywork.

Essentially, you are responsible for everything that happens within your Health Care business. Be smart. Be professional. Maintain whatever sets your business apart from others. Communicate effectively, and be attentive. Listen to what others have to say, and wisely find ways to turn all criticism into constructive ideas to promote the growth of your Health Care business. Ultimately, keep your vision and goals at the forefront while working harder each day to make sure that you are able to be at the top. At the end of the day, you will see the success that you may have once thought was unimaginable.

As a Health Care professional seeking to start a business, your choices are numerous. You can make any choice that you are passionate about, and in addition you can be success- ful. For more information about career alternatives, please visit www.BrilliantHealthCareGroup.com or e-mail info@ BrilliantHealthCareGroup.com.

# CHAPTER 15

BEFORE YOU START: YOUR BUSINESS CHECKLIST

**You were placed on this earth to achieve
your greatest self—to live out your
purpose and to do it courageously.**
—*DR. STEVE MARABOLI*

## 1. Determine viability.

B e brutally honest. Your start-up needs to be something you can make a profit doing or delivering. Ask yourself: would you buy it? Run the numbers: will customers pay enough so that you can cover costs and make a profit? Here is a list of twenty-nine more questions and tasks, attributed to noted investor Paul Graham.

## 2. Create a business plan.

It's easy to convince yourself that you don't need a business plan, but creating a business plan with financial projections forces you to think through the details. Keep your plan a living, breathing thing that you revisit and adapt regularly. Your business needs a plan to reach its destination. Without a business plan, you do not have a clear guide as to where you want to go.

## 3. Figure out the money.

Most start-ups take a lot more time to get off the ground than you expect. Know where your living expenses for the first year will come from. (Consider options including savings, a job, and spouse's income.) If you need financing for the business, start investigating as soon as possible.

## 4. Get family behind you.

Spend time making sure your spouse and other close family members buy into the concept of your start-up. You'll have enough challenges without resistance from family.

## 5. Choose a business name.

You want a name that will stick in your target audience's heads. And it shouldn't already be taken by another company. Do Google searches, and use a corporate name-search tool to see if the name you have in mind is unique. Check at the state and federal levels.

## 6. Register a domain name.

Get a domain name that matches your business name. A website with free hosting and a name like mysite.wordpress.com makes it seem like either (a) you are not running a real business or (b) you don't plan to be around long.

The more professionally you create your business, the more seriously your clients will take you.

## 7. Incorporate or figure out legal structure.

Incorporating your start-up can protect your personal assets. It is one of those "must haves." Decide about the best structure for your company (corporation, LLC, or sole proprietorship) with your attorney and accountant.

## 8. Apply for an EIN.

An Employer Identification Number (EIN) helps you separate yourself from your business. You'll need it if you plan to incorporate your business or open a business bank account. Plus, with an EIN you can avoid giving out your social-security number (an opening to identity theft). EIN numbers are free; apply online.

## 9. Investigate and apply for business licenses.

You may need a business license—if not several—for your startup, depending on your industry and where you are located. Most licenses are at the state or local level. Here in the United States, the Small Business Administration (SBA) has a helpful business license and permits tool.

## 10. Set up a website with an "about me" page.

Get your website up and running as soon as possible. Today it's necessary for credibility. Even if your product is not yet built, you can put company information on your website. Pages that give information about your company ("about me," "about us," or "contact us") are necessary on your website. Consumers can go to those pages to read about the main purpose and the vision of your business.

## 11. Register social-media profiles.

Getting set up on the major social-media channels (Facebook, LinkedIn, Twitter, and Instagram to start) will make marketing on them easier when you are ready to do so. It's also important to reserve your brand as a profile name. Try KnowEm.com to reserve the names.

## 12. Start your revenue stream.

Start generating revenue as soon as possible. In the early stages of a start-up, there is never enough money; resist the temptation to wait until things seem perfect. Remember too to have your lawyer create any customer contract forms necessary.

## 13. Rent retail or office space only if necessary.

If you are planning a brick-and-mortar business, you will need to address the issue of space early on. If you plan to run a retail business, pay attention to foot traffic, accessibility, and other factors that will affect the number of people who will walk in your store. *Exception*: If you don't have a brick-and-mortar or retail business, then wait to rent an office as long as possible to avoid saddling your start-up with lease payments.

## 14. Order business cards.

As a start-up founder, you'll be doing a lot of networking, so order plenty of business cards. They are inexpensive enough that you can reorder them later if any information changes. Without cards you lack credibility. I highly recommend Vistaprint.

## 15. Open a business bank account.

It's all too easy to use your personal bank account to pay for business expenses, but it becomes a gnarl to untangle later.

## 16. Set up your accounting system.

Once you have your bank account set up, choose an accounting program. Start keeping records in that system from the beginning of your venture. Few things will doom your business faster than books that are a mess.

## 17. Assign responsibilities to cofounders.

If you have one or more cofounders, it's imperative that you decide who will do what up front. Ensure that your decisions are placed in writing. Cofounder disagreements can destroy your business.

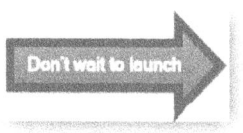 What You Can Do a Bit Later

While you don't want to put off these tasks
too long, they don't need to be checked
off your list before you launch.

## 18. Upgrade your smartphone and choose apps.

As an entrepreneur you are going to be on the go—a lot. I can't emphasize enough how useful a quality phone with good business apps can be in running your start-up. Get a credit-card swipe device to accept payments, too. I have several credit-card swipes, and I ensure that they are always working and ready to go. Apps are essential for creating postings, fliers, and business announcements as well as a wide array of business launching materials.

### 19. Find free advice.
Your local SBA office, SCORE, and other small-business resources can provide you with free advice, access to business templates, and other tools. Attend free workshops, webinars, and teleseminars.

### 20. Consult your insurance agent, and secure coverage.
Depending on the type of business you're starting, you may need insurance of one kind or another—including liability, workers' comp, and health insurance—especially if you hire full-time staff.

### 21. Hire your first employee.
Depending on the type of business you have, you may need staff from day one (retail), or you may be able to outsource to free-lancers, interns, and third-party vendors for a while (service and tech businesses). Just remember, trying to do everything yourself takes you away from growing the business.

### 22. Line up suppliers and service providers.
Finding a good source of inventory is crucial, especially in certain types of businesses (retail, manufacturing). Beyond inventory, line up good, reliable suppliers and service providers so you don't have to sweat the details.

### 23. File for trademarks and patents.
The best thing to do is consult an attorney early about the need for patents, especially. Get the advice early. Then you may be able to defer filing for a while, depending on the nature of your business.

### 24. Work your network.

Reach out to former coworkers and colleagues, as well as friends and family. Don't pressure them to buy your products or services. Instead, tap into them as resources for introductions and for help with other things on this start-up checklist.

### 25. Don't waste too much time on partnerships.

Be careful about wasting time on business-partnership discussions. Your business won't be attractive to potential partners until you start making headway. Focus your precious time on making sales and getting customers.

### 26. Refine your pitch.

You need a good elevator pitch for many people: potential investors, customers, clients, prospective new hires, bankers. If you can't persuasively and clearly pitch your business, how can you expect key stakeholders to buy in?

### 27. Refine your product and marketing and sales approach.

As you go along, you will learn more about the marketplace. Use customer feedback to refine your product-and-service offerings and your marketing approach.

### 28. Secure your IT.

Whether you're running a tech company or not, you likely have sensitive data on computers and devices that you want protected. Protect it from intrusions and disasters. Back it up! IT problems can derail a fledgling company.

## 29. Get a salesperson or sales team in place.

In many start-ups the business owner starts out as the chief sales-person. But to grow you need someone dedicated solely to sales, so you can focus on activities other than day-to-day sales.

## 30. Hire a mentor/coach/consultant.

It's all too easy to work *in* your business rather than *on* it. As Michael Gerber tells us in his book *The E-Myth*, we need to be working *on* our businesses if we want them to grow and flourish. A mentor who has succeeded in your industry can provide you with priceless advice and serve as a sounding board.

It is very important that you seek a coach or a mentor who knows and understands your industry. Each industry is so specific. When I started out as a Health Care consultant, I quickly found out that not every coach or mentor understands the business of Health Care start-up. Many coaches will not admit their lack of savvy to their clients, but it's almost impossible for a coach without experience in your industry to help you clarify your mission and your calling. Seek a coach who knows your industry and has operational experience in it.

# SUMMARY

This book will change your life if you begin to apply the principles. I pray and trust that it will inspire you to greater heights as you travel your Health Care journey of entrepreneurship, touching and changing lives in many ways. In the end you are making a significant difference in others' lives, as well as adding value—which is the ultimate goal. Never be afraid to step outside of your comfort zone. In order for you to achieve greatness, you must be willing to take that mammoth leap of faith as well as a deep dive. You will never be the best that you can be if you don't take the risk. I like what Dr. Martin Luther King said: "Faith is taking the first step even though you don't see the whole staircase."

## Eva M. Francis, RN, MSN, CCRN
*Entrepreneur, Health Care Speaker, Executive Leadership & Business Coach, and Trainer*

Dedicated to providing training, insights, and strategies to advance your career and elevate you to another level and beyond.

Eva M. Francis, MSN, RN, CCRN is a former hospital and nurse executive who is now the president and founder of Brilliant Health Care Training & Consulting, Inc., V&E Health care Institute as well as CO-Founder of The Leaders Lead LLC.

Eva is the Founder of The National Nurse Empowerment Inc. which is a non profit organization serves to empower and inspire nurses & nurse leaders to elevate and achieve more in their career and in their life.

Eva is also a Health Care Influencer, Certified Leadership Coach and a Reinvention Strategist who helps Health Care professionals and leaders to examine organizational obstacles, break through barriers, and achieve more in their business and career by providing tools, strategies, and training to enhance and impact their brand—resulting in a higher bottom line. Eva Francis also empowers nurses and other allied Health Care professionals to serve, lead, and succeed in their career and business.

*Eva M. Francis is a certified leadership speaker, trainer, and leadership coach with The John Maxwell Team.*

www.ingramcontent.com/pod-product-compliance
Lightning Source LLC
Chambersburg PA
CBHW051335170526

45166CB00002B/826

9 7 8 1 5 2 2 8 6 2 1 8 5